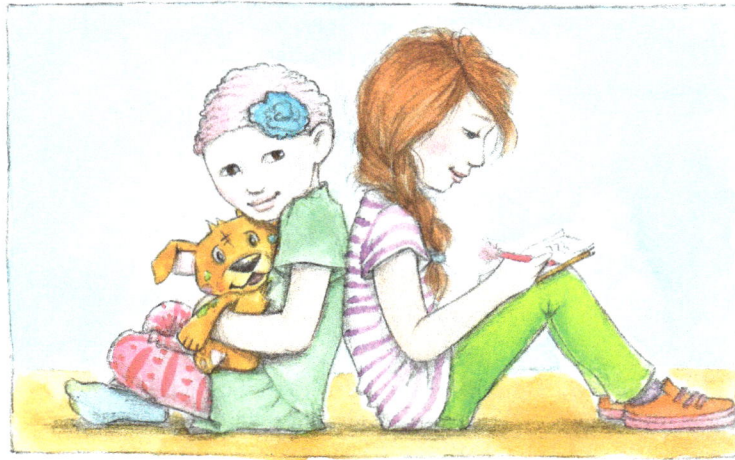

Jamie's Journey

Cancer from the Voice of a Sibling

by Sharon Wozny

illustrated by Melissa Bailey

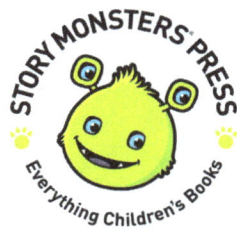

STORY MONSTERS PRESS
Everything Children's Books

Linda F. Radke, Publisher
Story Monsters Press
An imprint of Story Monsters LLC
4696 W. Tyson Street
Chandler, AZ 85226
480-940-8182
Publisher@storymonsters.com
www.StoryMonstersPress.com

www.jamiesjourneybook.com

Printed in the United States of America

Illustrator: Melissa Bailey
Cover Design & Page Layout: Jeff Yesh & Kris Taft Miller
Editor: Conrad J. Storad
Proofreader: Cristy Bertini
Project Manager: Diane Timmons

Thank you very much to Jeff Luttrell for providing the art inspiration for the character of Speckles.

Publisher's Cataloging-In-Publication Data
Names: Wozny, Sharon, author. | Bailey, Melissa, 1978- illustrator.
Title: Jamie's journey : cancer from the voice of a sibling / by Sharon Wozny ; illustrated by Melissa Bailey.
Description: [Second edition]. | [Chandler, Arizona] : Story Monsters Press, [2025] | Interest age level: 005-014. | Summary: The first half of the book is about 13-year-old Jamie who describes the roller coaster of emotions she experiences when her 10-year-old sister, Jordan, is diagnosed with cancer. Jamie laments the loss of her normal teenage life and describes feeling forgotten as her family focuses on Jordan's medical needs. Jamie finds solace through journaling about her experience, and encourages the reader to write about his or her own journey on the pages provided in the
[second half of the] book.--Publisher.
Identifiers: ISBN: 9781589854024 (paperback) | 9781589854031 (ebook)
Subjects: LCSH: Cancer in children--Psychological aspects--Juvenile fiction. | Cancer in children--Patients--Family relationships--Juvenile fiction. | Sisters--Juvenile fiction. | Teenage girls--Diaries--Juvenile fiction. | CYAC: Cancer--Psychological aspects--Fiction. | Sisters--Fiction. | Teenage girls--Diaries--Fiction.
Classification: LCC: PZ7.1.W69 Ja 2025 | DDC: [Fic]--dc23

---

www.StoryMonstersPress.com

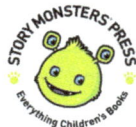

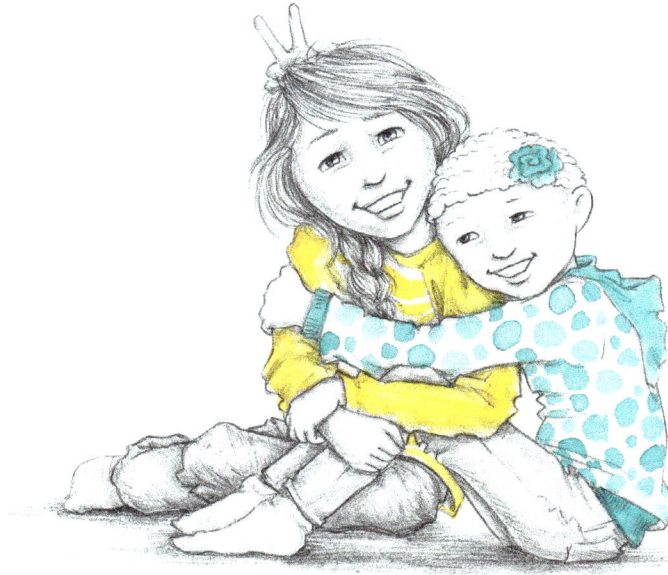

Dedicated to the siblings of cancer patients everywhere!

I thank God every day for bringing Children's Cancer Network (CCN) into my life; the families who I have met through my volunteer work are the inspiration for this book. CCN focuses on the whole family through their child's cancer diagnosis with programs and services that celebrate each member of the family.

The siblings of cancer patients have a road to travel which they do with love, compassion, and selflessness.

You are the unsung heroes! You are all survivors!

—Sharon

xoxo

To Grandma B. and Grandma S.

—Melissa

No Matter the Language...

Sibling: One or more individuals having a parent in common; a brother or sister

Special: Especially important or loved

Love: Strong affection arising out of kinship for another

Friend: A person who helps or supports someone or something

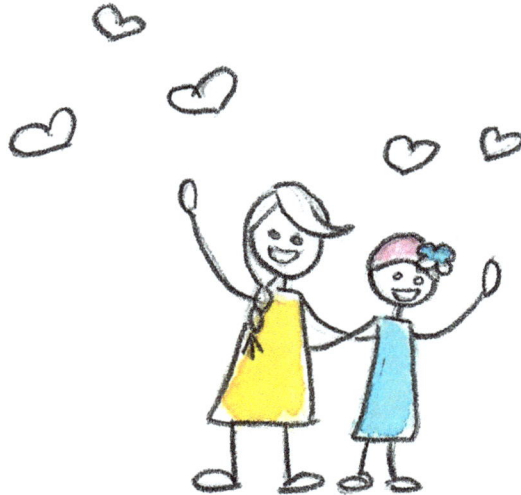

"It's important that we share our experiences with other people. Your story will heal you and your story will heal somebody else. When you tell your story, you free yourself and give other people permission to acknowledge their own story."

—Iyanla Vanzant

As you read each page of our story, think about yours!

This is our story...

Hi! My name is Jamie. I'm thirteen years old. I'm in the eighth grade. My sister Jordan is ten years old. She's a fifth grader.

The fact that this book is in your hands means you're on the road to healing. You see, I'm just like you. I'm the sibling of a cancer survivor.

I get it. I've ridden the emotional roller coaster. One day you think you're fine. The next moment, feelings you never thought you could have are threatening to explode!

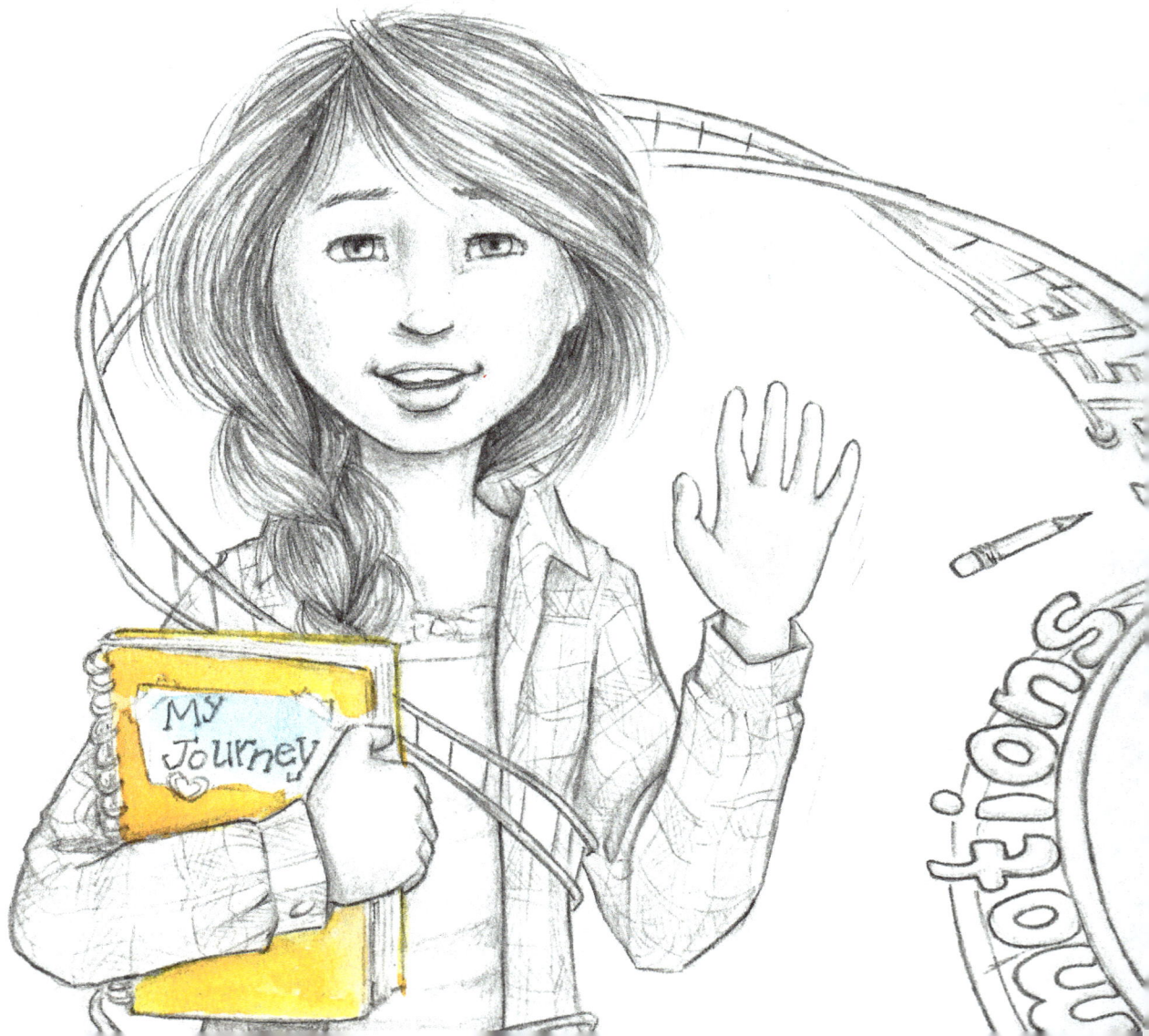

Our life was normal. We were going to sleepovers, hanging at the mall, shopping. We had softball practice and dance lessons. You know what I mean, fun stuff.

But then Jordan started having headaches. She had them for more than a week, off and on. She was just so tired. Much more than an active ten-year-old girl should have been.

Our parents made an appointment with the pediatrician. What we thought was going to be one visit to the doctor turned into a bunch of appointments.

First they did blood work. Then Jordan had to have a CT scan. The next day, she had an MRI at the children's hospital. CT scans and MRI's are ways for doctors to take pictures of the inside of a person's body. The doctors wanted to know more about what was making Jordan sick so they could help her get better.

Our family waited for an hour to find out the results. Finally, the doctor entered the room. That is when everything changed.

The doctor explained the test results to us. He said the tests showed that Jordan had a brain tumor. Before we knew it, he said the C word . . . cancer!

Life as we knew it was turned upside down.

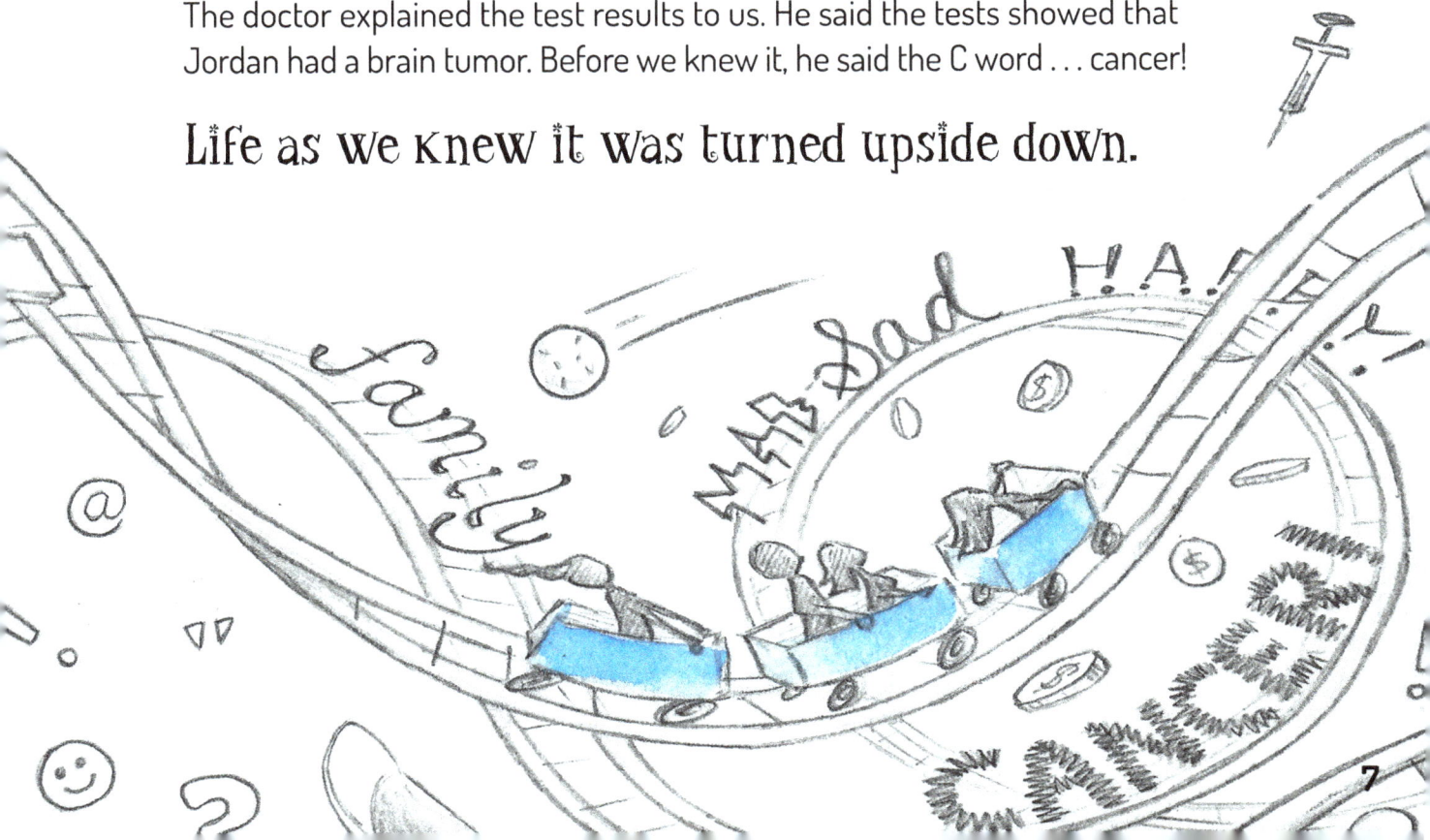

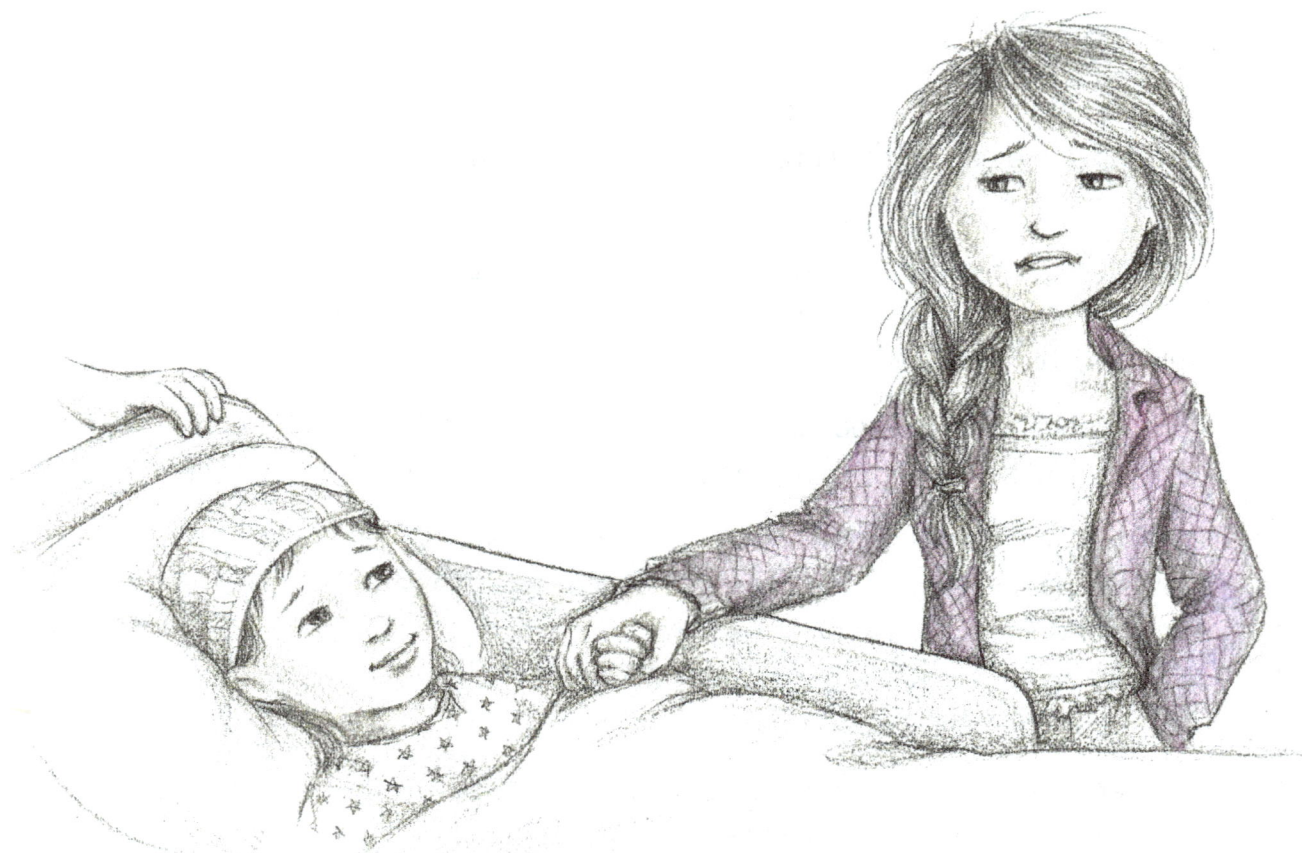

The doctors scheduled surgery for Jordan. Everything seemed to happen quickly. It was all such a blur. I really didn't have time to think about everything.

I watched as a nurse wheeled Jordan into the operating room. My heart felt like it almost stopped.

What would happen? Would my baby sister be all right? Would the doctors be able to remove the entire tumor? Would she be the same when the operation was over?

I was very worried.

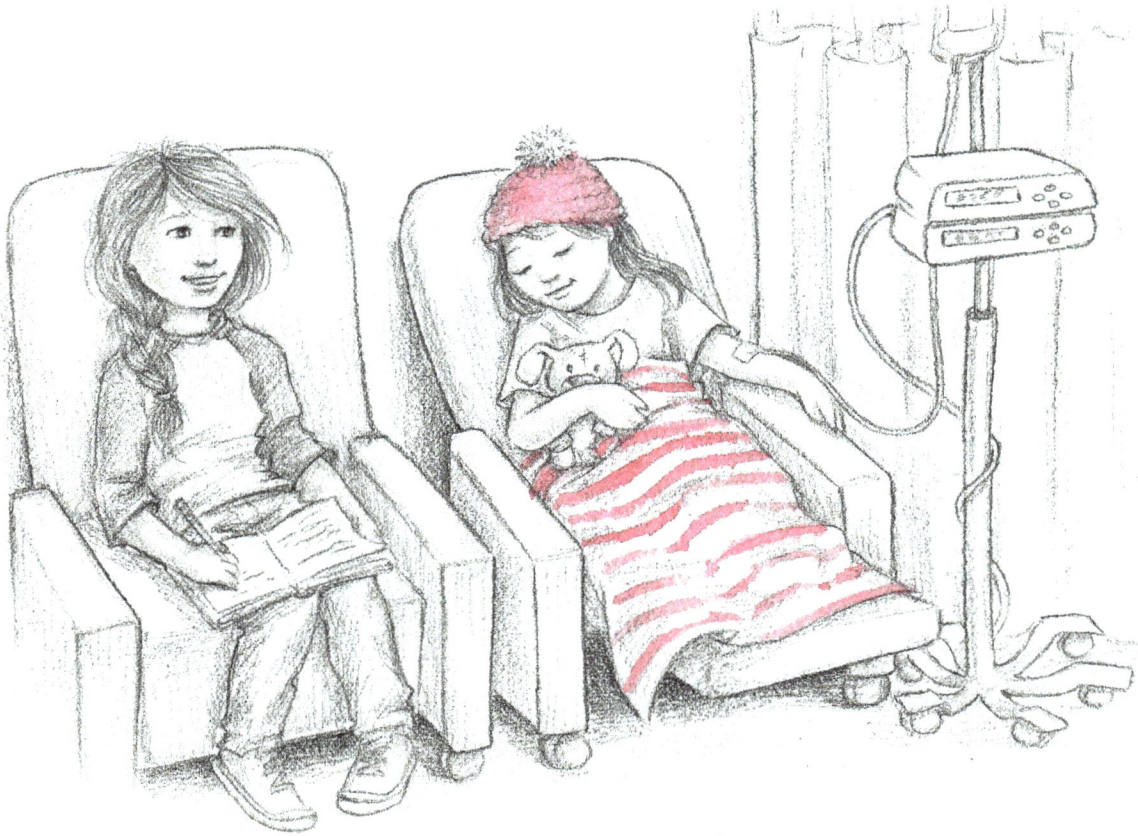

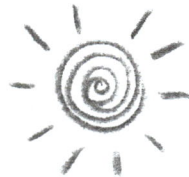

Jordan's surgery was a success.

The surgeon removed every bit of the tumor.

Now, my little sister's long road to recovery would begin. Her treatment plan started in the hospital. She had to have chemotherapy, or chemo, which is special medicine that slows down or stops the cancer cells in your body. Jordan would have to stay in the hospital for six weeks.

At this moment, I was relieved.

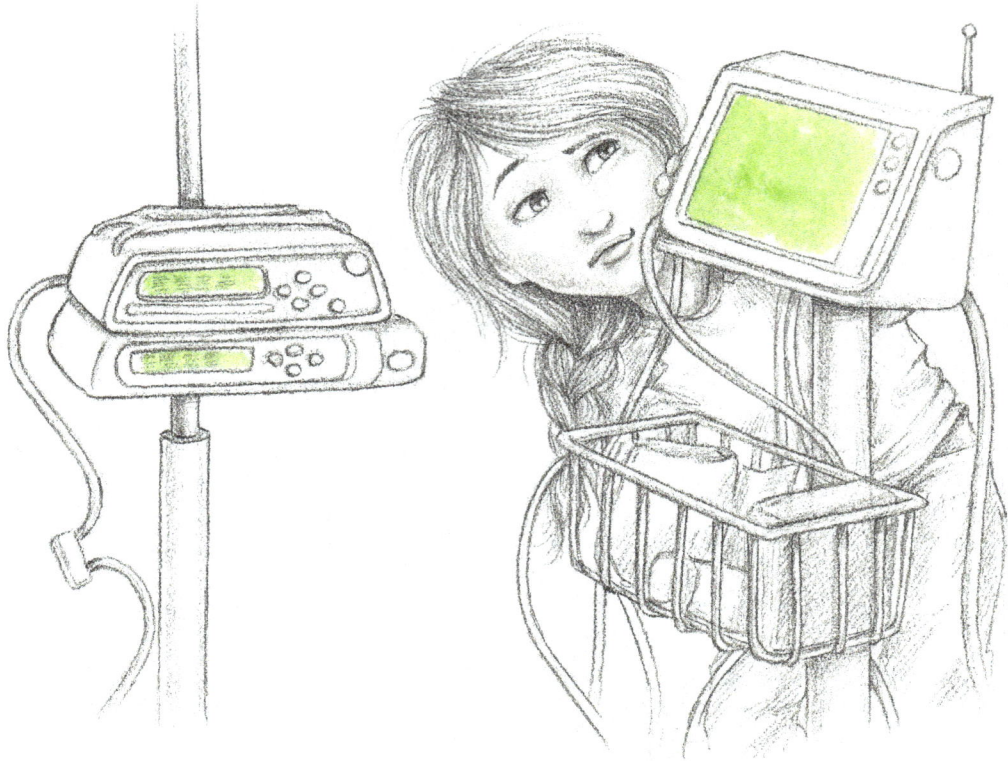

The nurses and doctors kept coming in and out of my sister's room. They always disinfected their hands. Sometimes they put on a mask and gown.

Jordan knew what was coming.

"Pokes." That's what they called it.

Pokes meant they stuck Jordan with needles. Then they hooked her up to IVs which delivered the medicine. There were plenty of other machines in the room as well. One monitored my sister's heart rate. Another kept track of her blood pressure. Another listed her temperature.

What did all of the numbers mean?

I listened to everyone. I began to ask questions.

I was curious.

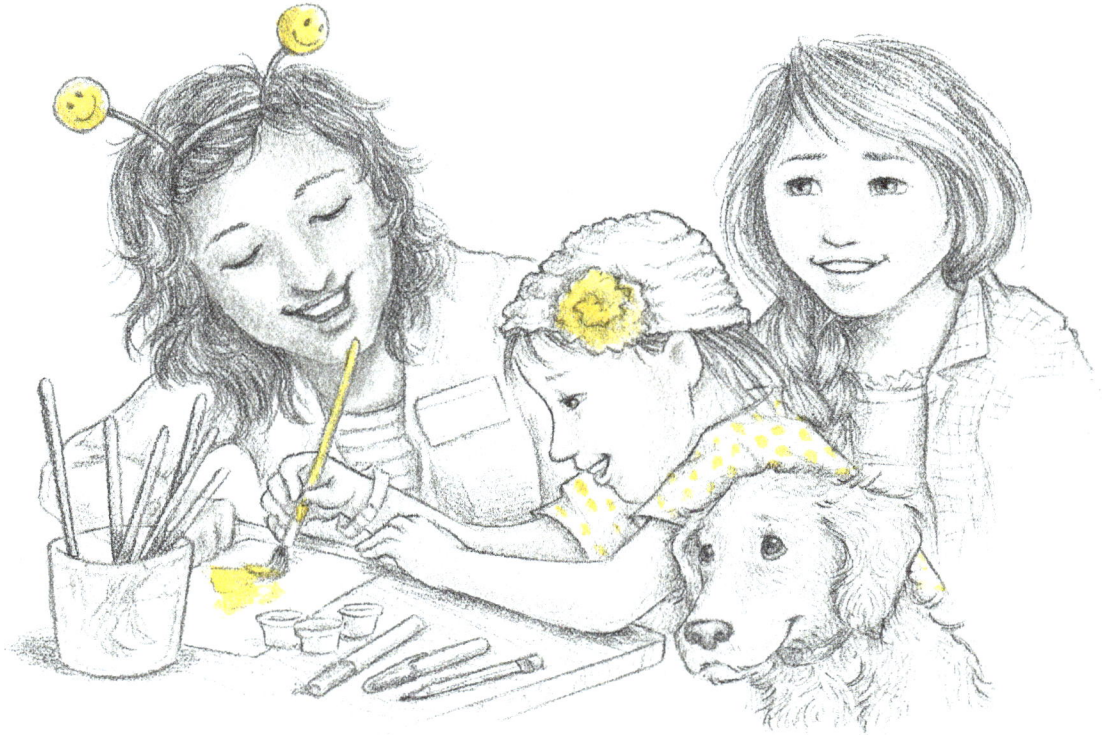

Lots of people came in and out of my sister's room. Not all of them were doctors or nurses. Child life specialists and child life assistants visited.

I thought of them as angels here on earth, because I saw Jordan smile when they opened the door. Each one of them brightened Jordan's day with smiles, encouragement, and love.

Whenever Jordan saw them, she knew something fun was coming. Sometimes it was an arts and crafts project. Or it might be a visit from a therapy dog ready to give love. A few times it was a visit from a local sports star.

Most of the time, it was simply an invitation to come to the playroom for extra special activities.

The best part was that the family could also attend.

I was happy!

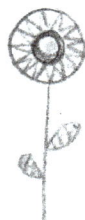

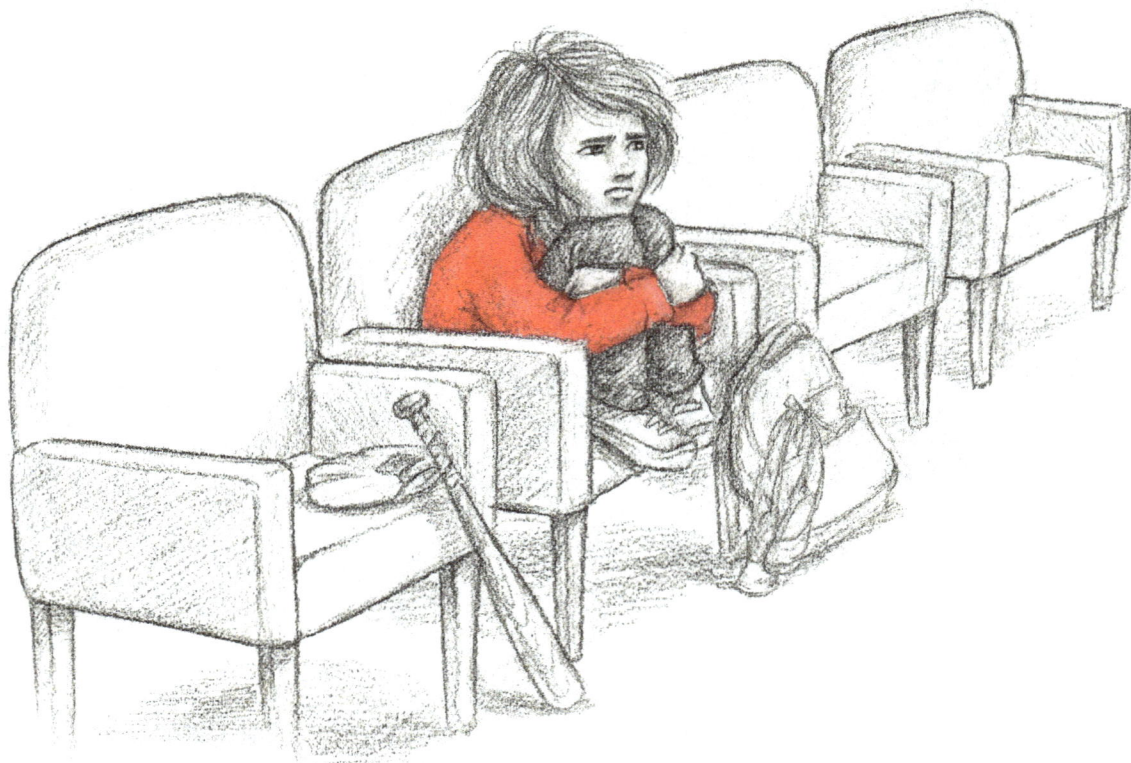

After six weeks in the hospital, Jordan was allowed to come home. But she still needed to go to the outpatient clinic once a week for her chemotherapy.

Sometimes these appointments went on schedule. But other times, an hour visit often turned into five hours. This seemed to happen more often than I wanted.

When it did, I had to miss my dance class or softball practice.

It just didn't seem fair.

I was angry.

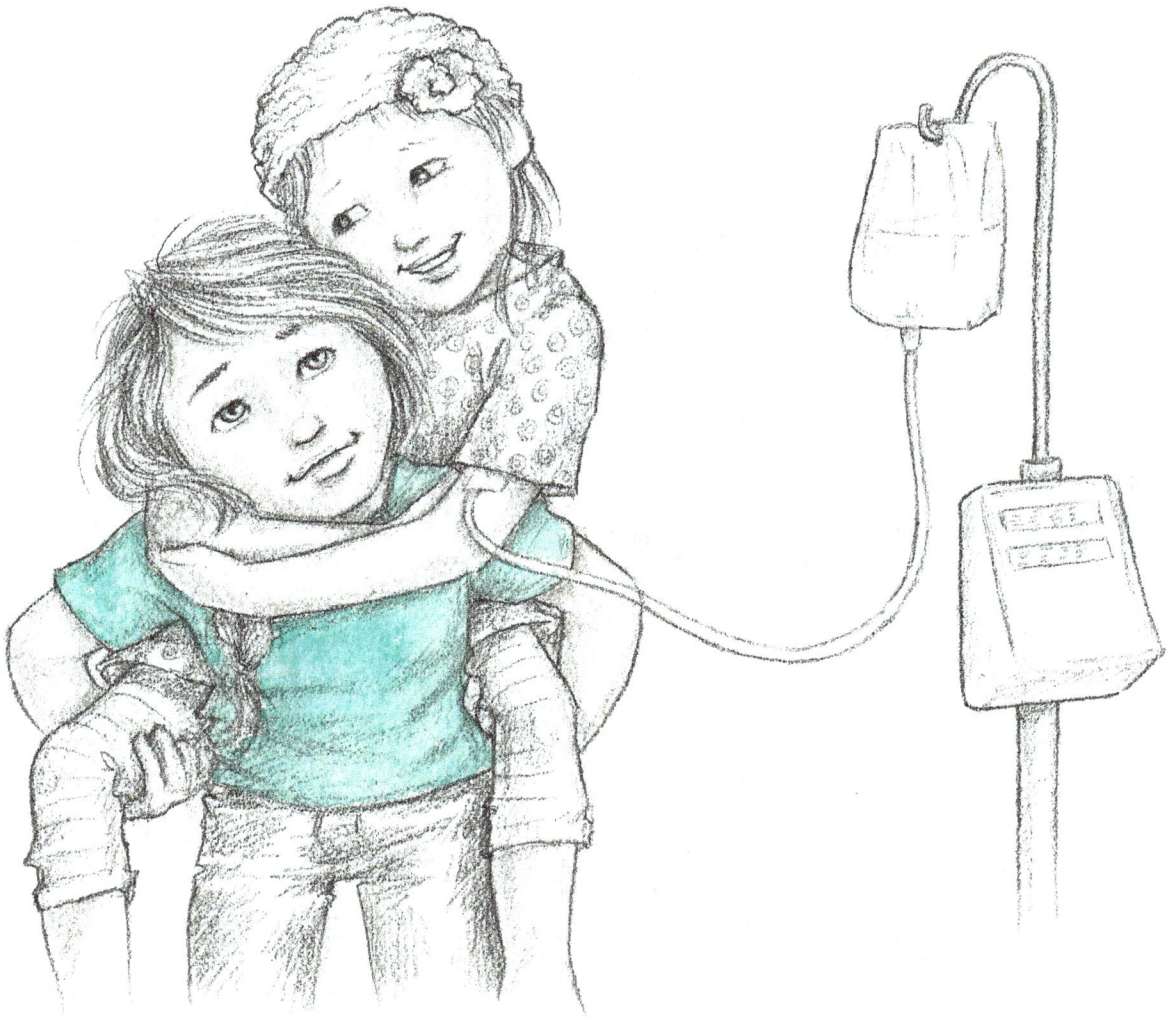

Sometimes I think about all the powerful medicine that was pumped into Jordan's body. You know what? I am blown away with the way she handled it all.

Jordan did it with a smile and a totally positive attitude.

I was proud to be her big sister.

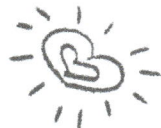

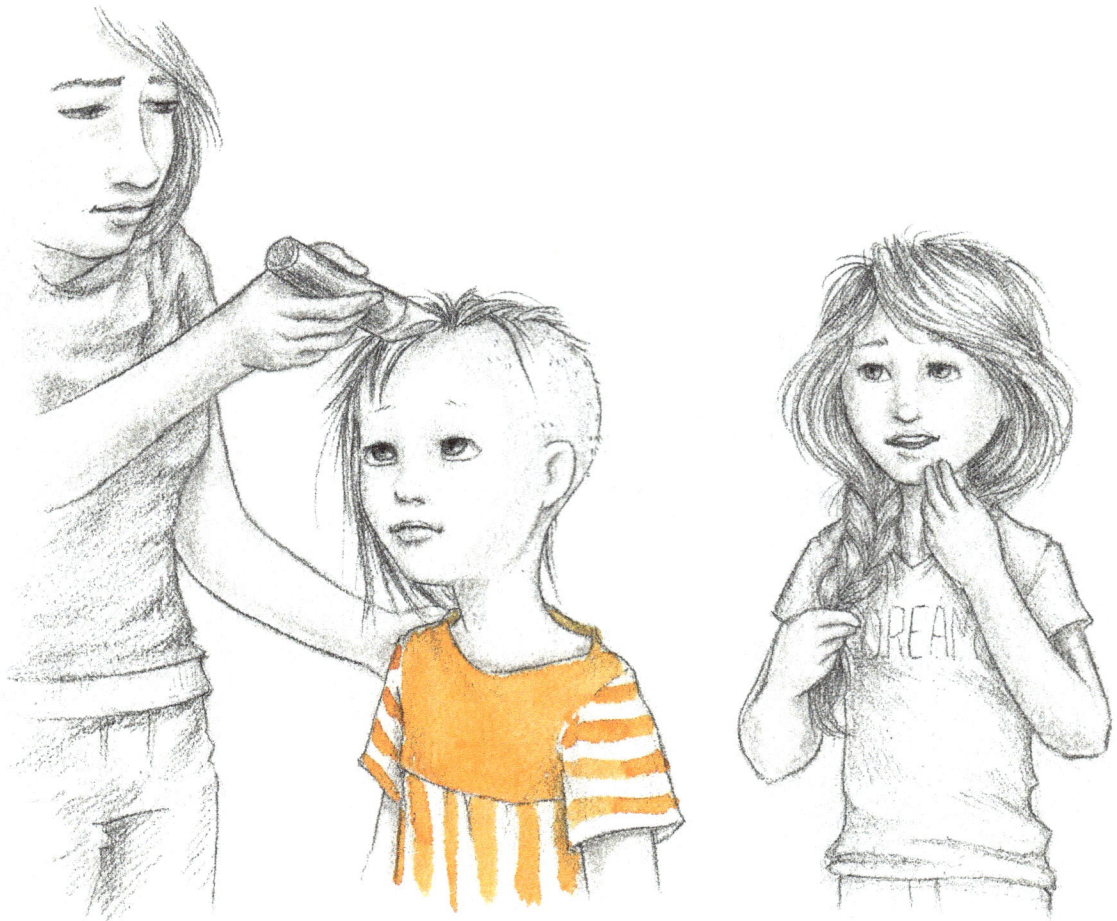

It wasn't long after Jordan began her chemotherapy that her hair began to fall out. There were lots of tears. And there were jokes.

Finally, Jordan made the decision to just shave it all off. That would be much better than waiting to find clumps of hair on the pillow every morning.

Bald is beautiful!

It was such a brave decision!

Could I have been that brave?

I was inspired!

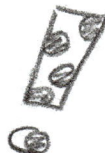

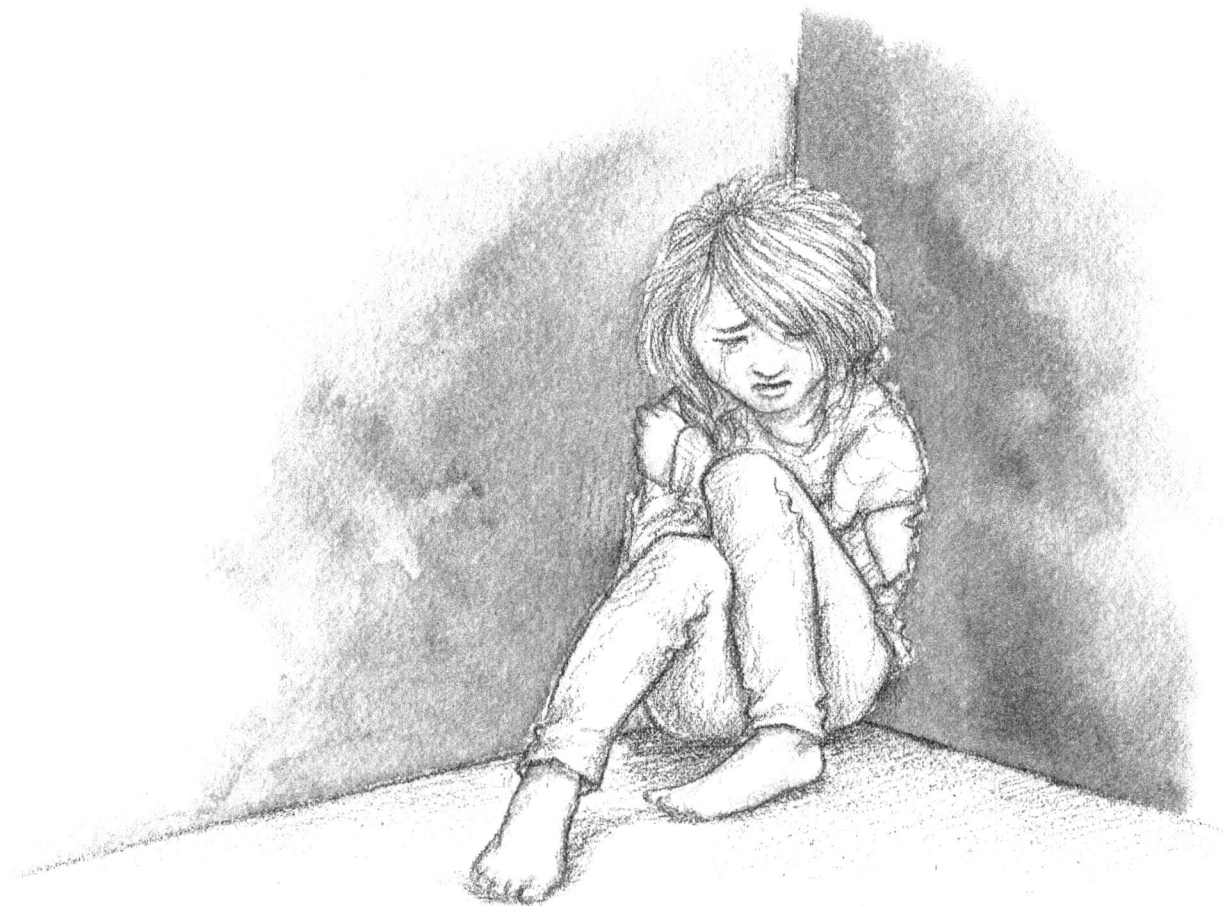

The lives of everyone in my family changed. Those changes seemed to come faster and faster.

My parents were wrapped up in Jordan's appointments. They worried if the chemo was working. Would she need more surgery? They were always watching her.

Of course, so did I. But I also started to wonder if I even mattered to my parents anymore. I cried hard sometimes, almost uncontrollably.

I had such darkness in my heart that it scared me.

I was feeling forgotten.

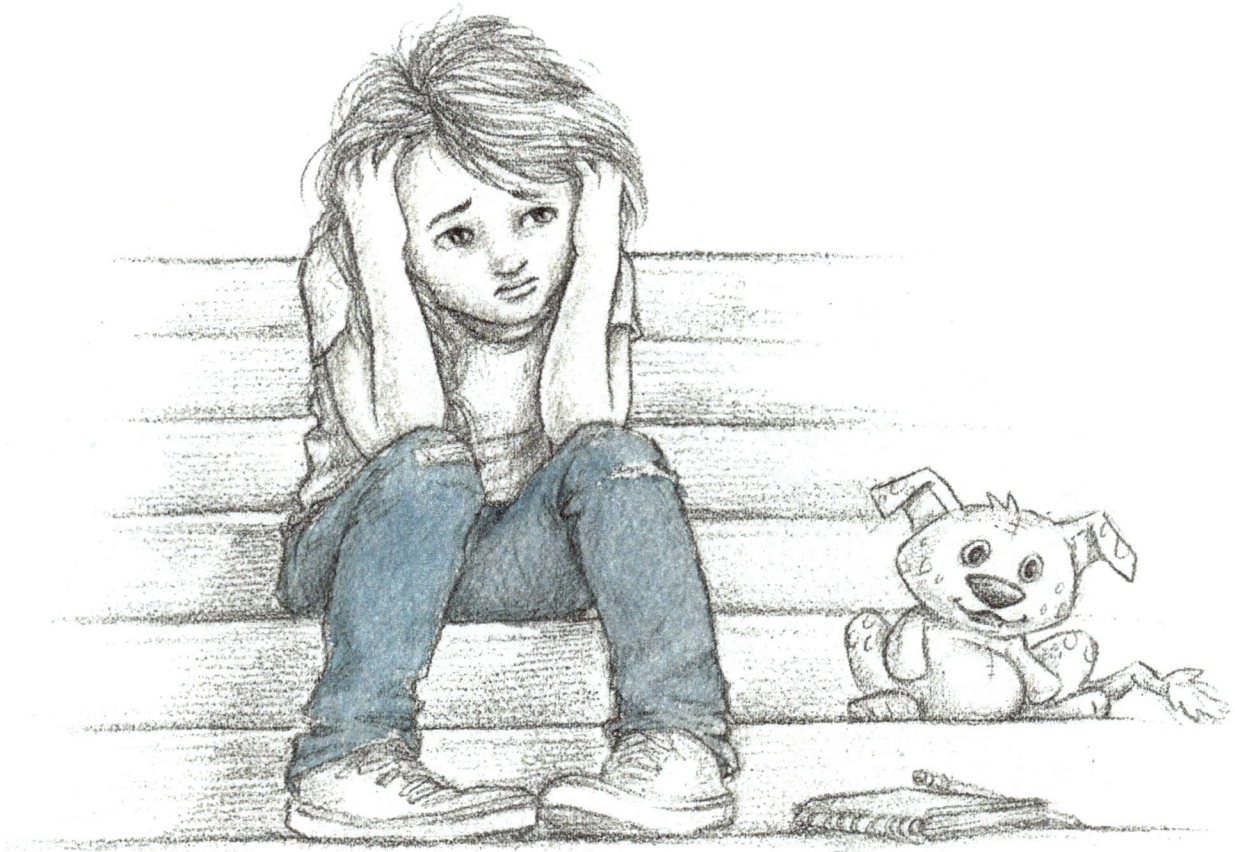

Unknown feelings started to fill my heart.

I felt anger. I felt fear.

I was worried. I felt jealous.

Was this normal? Did other siblings feel this way?

My friends didn't understand. How could they?
Their little sisters didn't have cancer. Mine did.

I didn't want to bother my parents and talk about my
feelings. They had plenty to deal with taking care of Jordan.
I needed to be strong.

But I was confused.

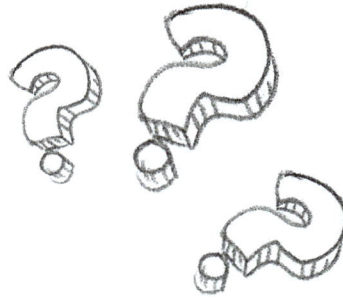

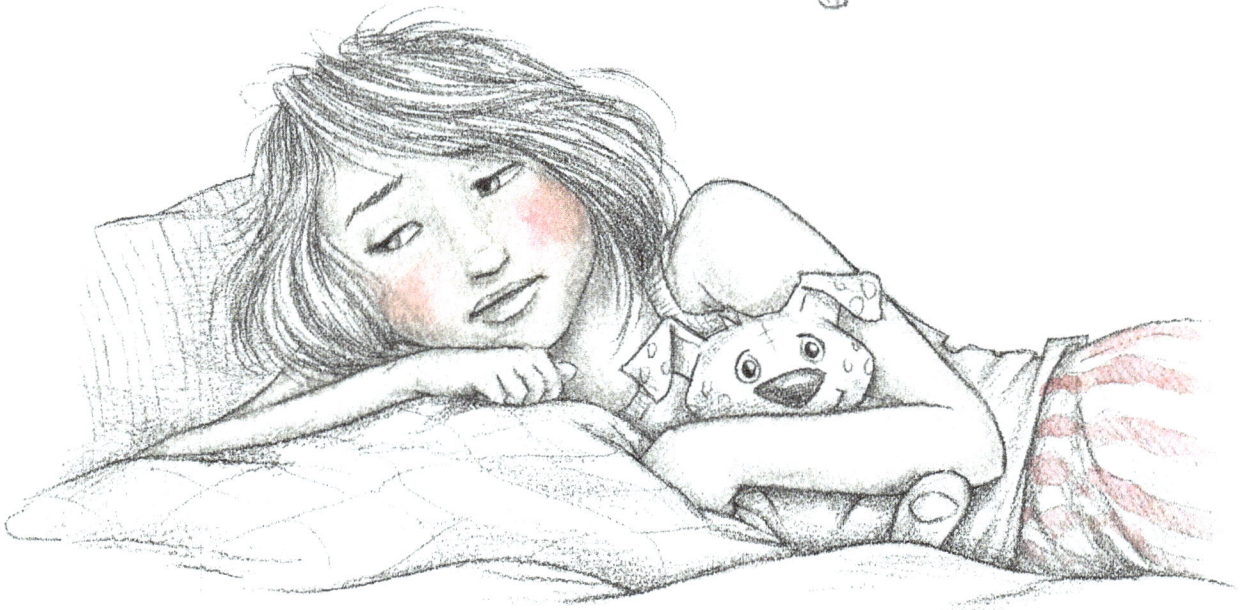

I kept thinking . . . why *my* sister?

Would I catch this cancer?

Was it okay for me to have fun when Jordan was sick?

Why *not* me?

Would my friends still want to come over to our house?

I was feeling guilty.

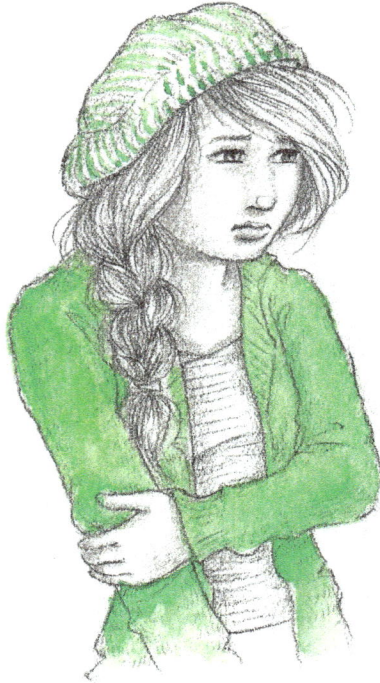

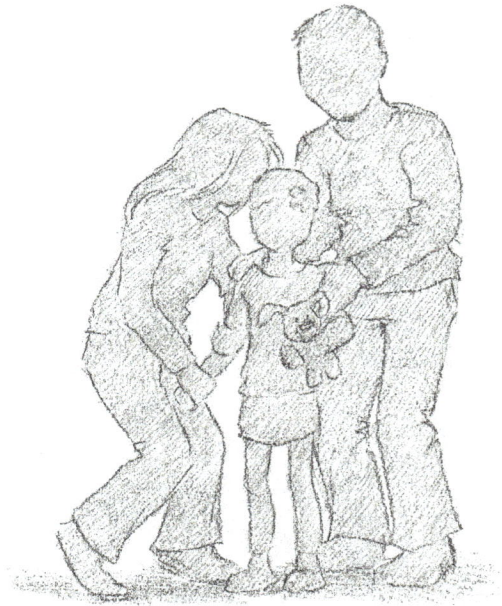

Okay, I admit it, I like attention.

Before all this happened with Jordan, everything was pretty equal.
Both of us received compliments on our individual achievements.
But now, it seemed as if nobody wanted to know about me anymore.

Everywhere we went, Jordan got *all* the attention!

Jordan got presents and free trips. Jordan got sympathy.
Jordan seemed to get every minute of our parents' time.

She didn't have to do chores. She got to watch TV all the time.
And she had lots of new toys.

Basically, Jordan was being treated like a "rock star" just because
she had cancer.

Did that mean I needed to be ignored? I didn't ask *not* to get cancer.

I've made sacrifices. I knew I shouldn't feel this way.

I was jealous!

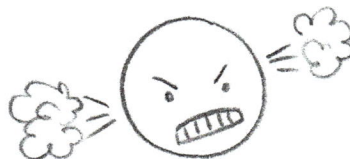

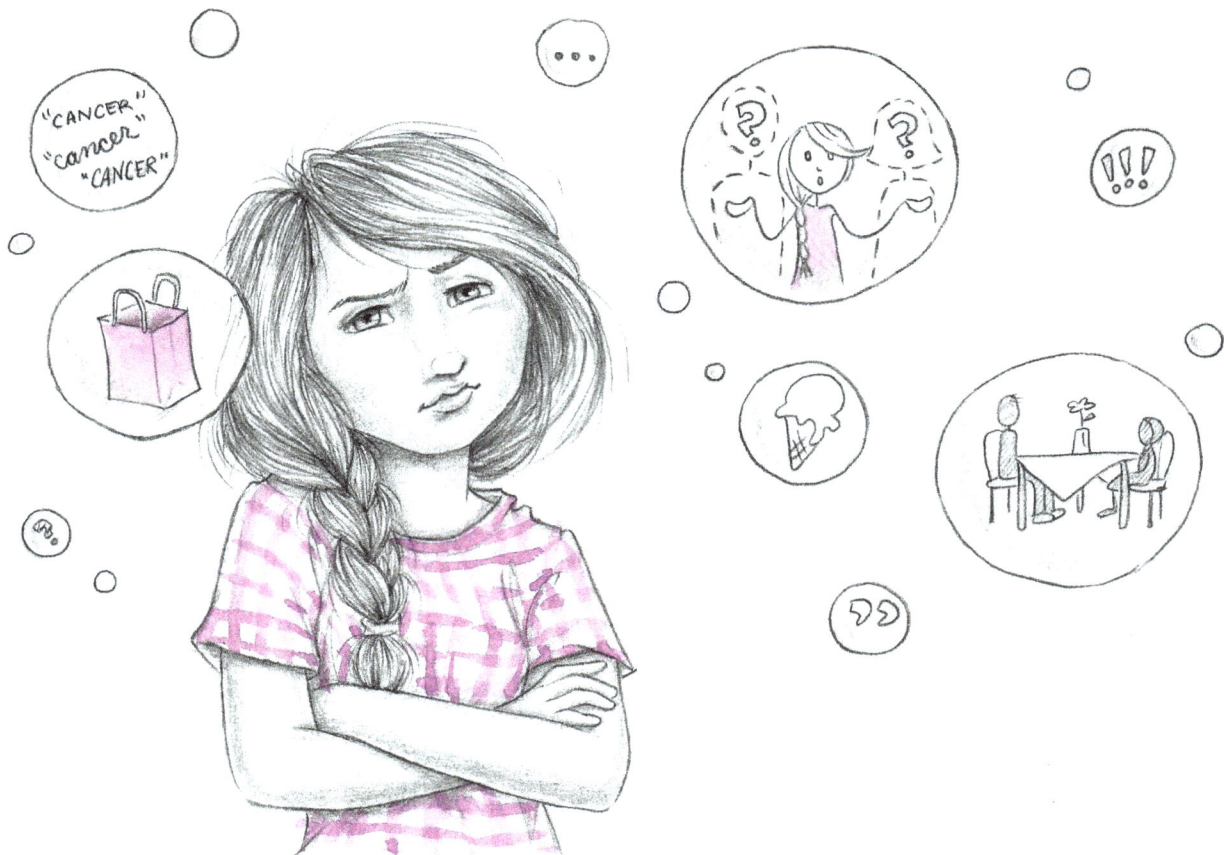

Did you ever feel like you lost your parents? I did.

My mom and dad were exhausted!

Cancer talk was everywhere. Even when we didn't talk about it, I knew they were thinking all about it.

I rarely got any alone time with them.

My date nights with my dad were a thing of the past.

Mom and I didn't even have time for shopping and ice cream anymore.

I was feeling selfish.

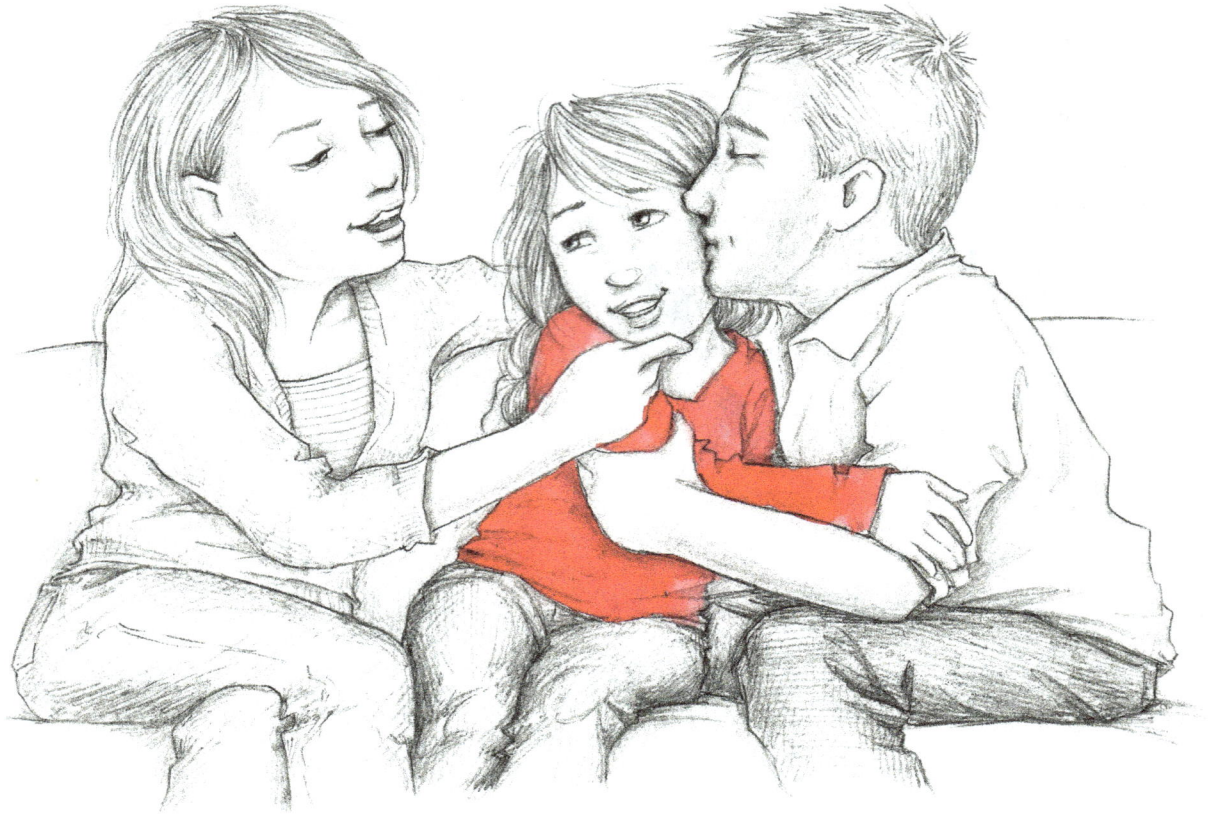

Deep down, I knew my parents still loved me. And I knew in my heart that Jordan needed more attention.

One night, after Jordan had gone to bed, my parents sat down with me on the couch.

They both held me tight. They told me they knew how hard my sister's battle with cancer had been on me.

They said they hadn't forgotten about me.

They told me how extremely proud they were of the way I had handled all of the huge changes in our lives.

I was feeling loved and valued.

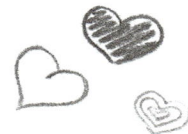

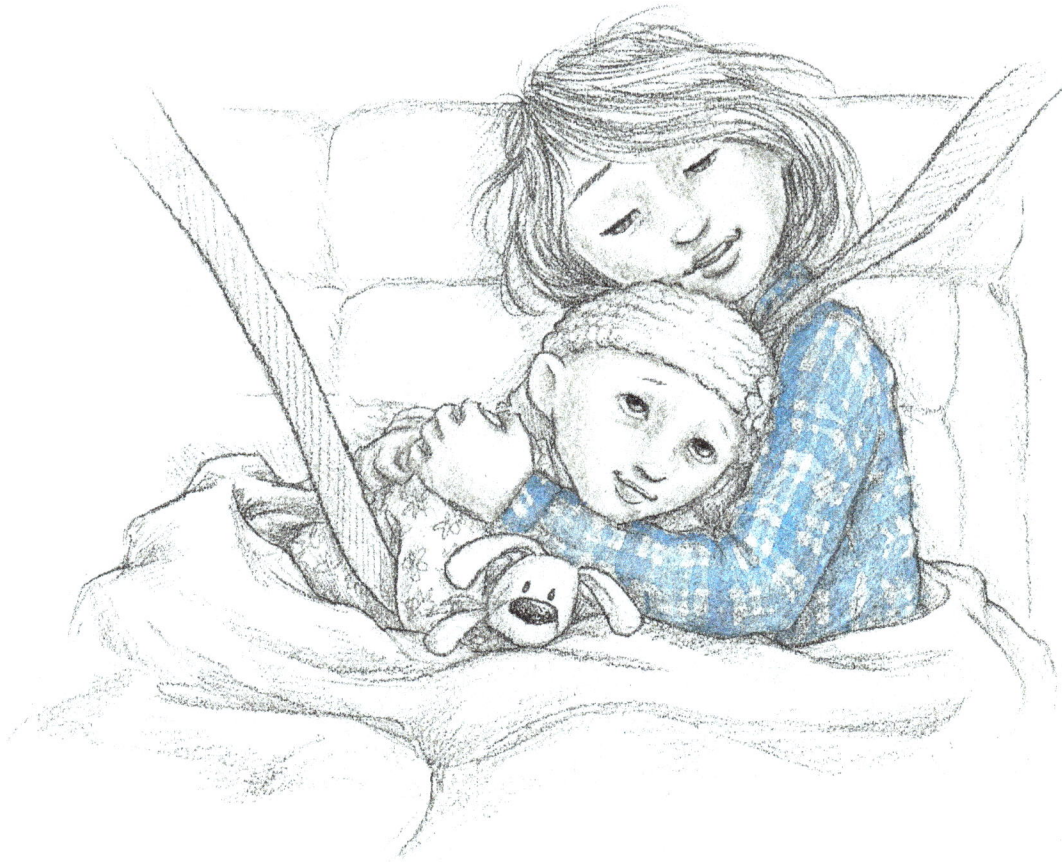

There were lots of tough days and nights in the months that followed.

There were many trips to hospital.

One late night sticks in my memory. Jordan had a very high fever. We all piled into the car and drove her to the emergency room.

I cuddled with my sister in the back seat. We were wrapped in a blanket and had her favorite stuffed dog wedged between us. Jordan smiled and settled in closer.

I remember whispering, "I am here, just hold on tight."

I felt helpful.

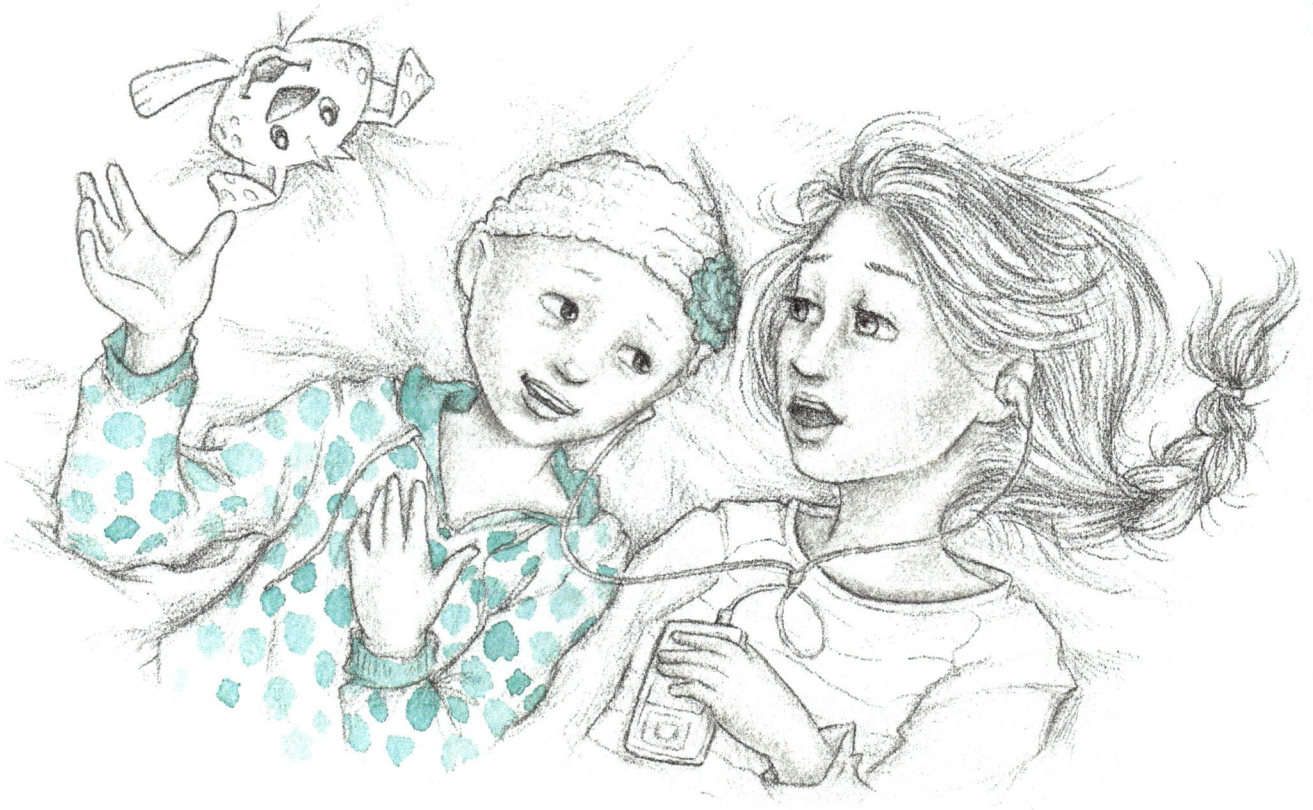

I remember another special day. It was almost a year after this emotional roller coaster had started its wild ride.

Jordan and I were hanging out in her room listening to music. She told me that I was her hero.

She told me that without my love, she wouldn't have been able to fight her cancer.

Then Jordan actually apologized to *me* for having cancer. She said she was sorry for hogging all of our parents' attention.

She said she was sorry that we were not able to do all the things we used to do together.

And she told me she was sorry that I had to miss *my* activities!

I was speechless.

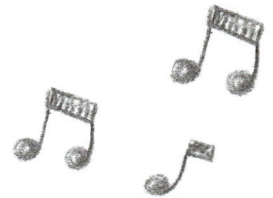

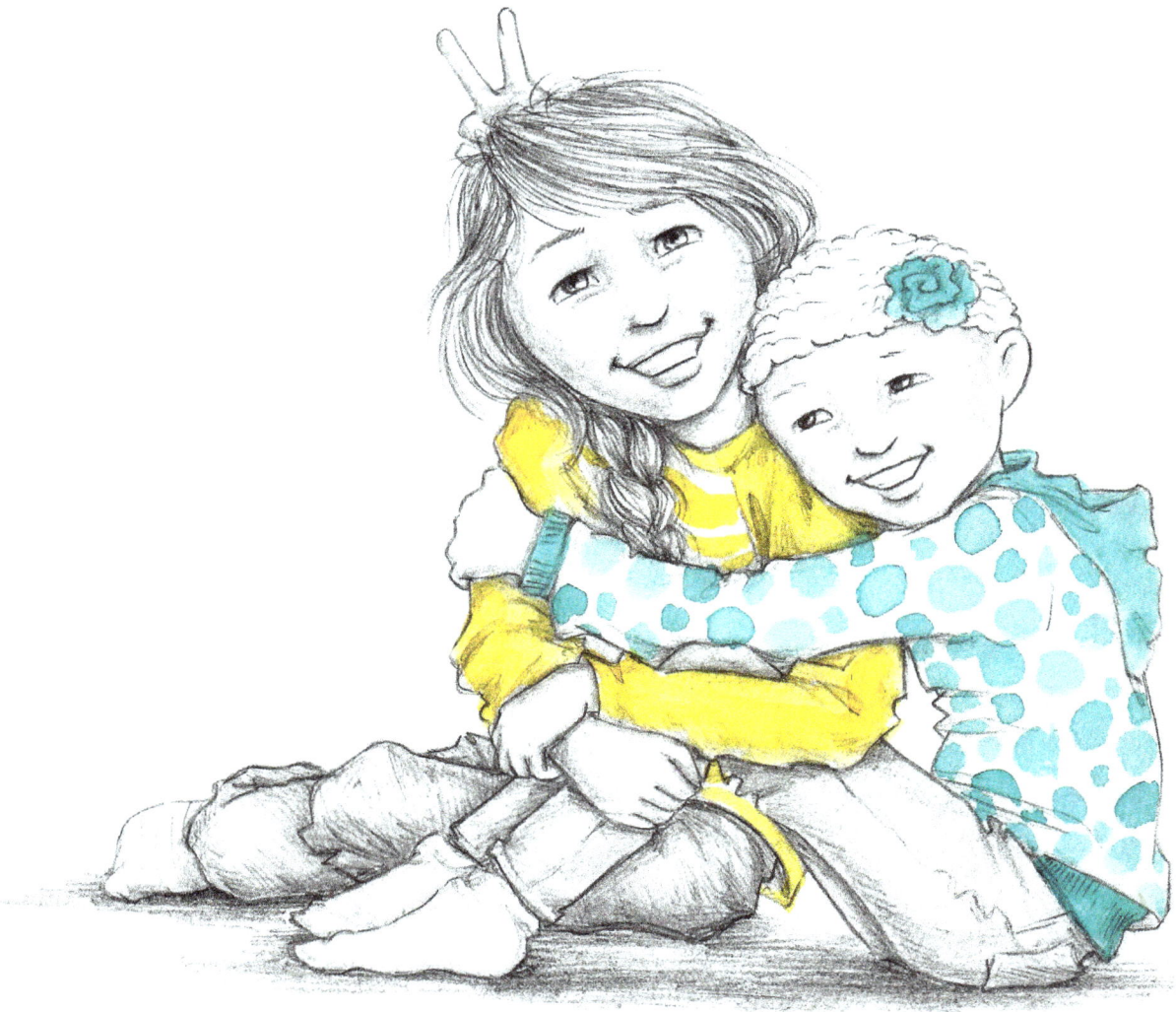

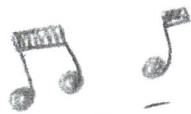

One of our favorite songs was playing.

Right then I knew that the emotional
roller coaster had come full circle!

I hugged Jordan with all my love.

I was happy again.

AFTERWORD

Remember how I said I had darkness in my heart? You know I really didn't, any more than you may feel you have in your heart.

What we really hate is CANCER.

Cancer affects everyone and everything!

Cancer makes life all topsy-turvy. It's a roller coaster that is not very fun at all. Just remember we are never forgotten. Instead, know that we are loved and treasured. We are sibling survivors!

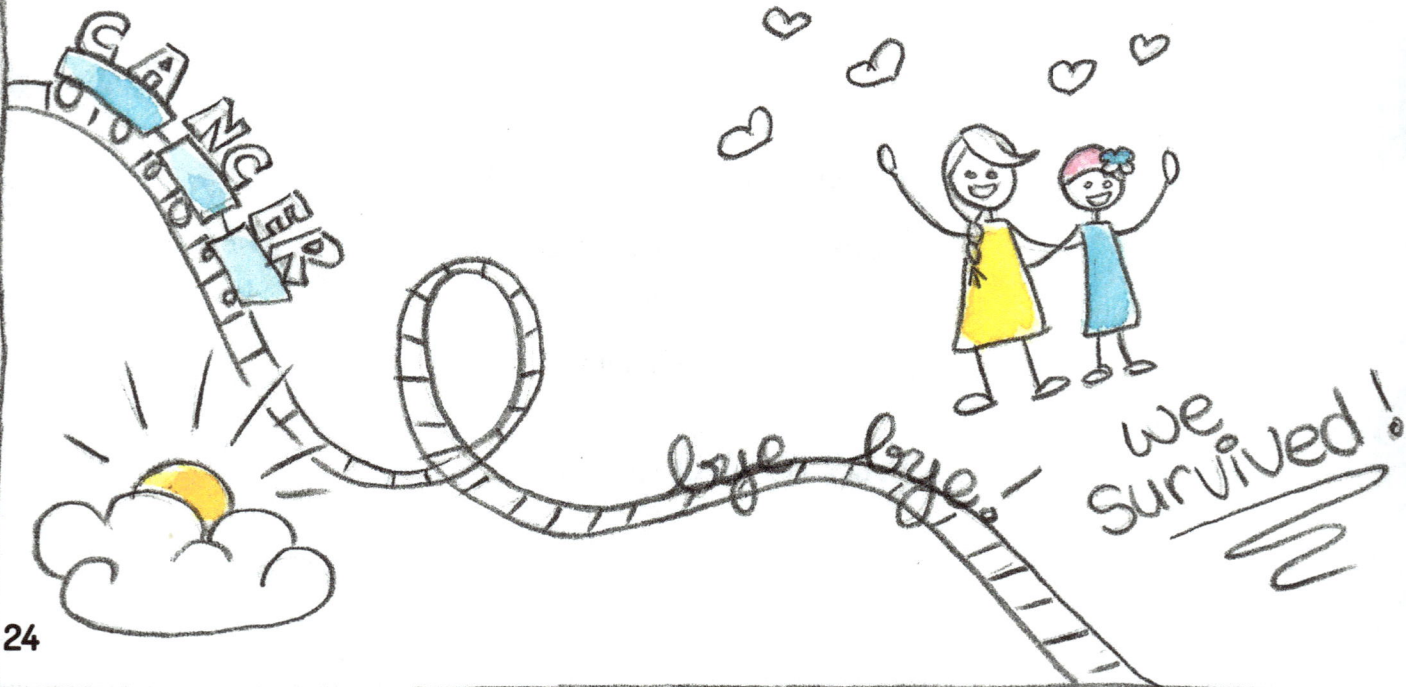

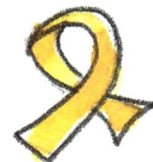

Don't forget that there are places to go and people you can call for help. You don't have to travel this sibling role on your own.

Here are some sites you can check out for more information:

- www.alexslemonade.org
- www.cancer.org
- www.childrenscancernetwork.org
- www.childcancer.org.nz

Remember, the child life specialists and social workers at your hospital are always there for you, too. They can put you in touch with resources and local organizations.

Love,

Jamie

xoxo

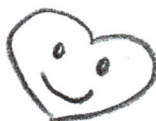

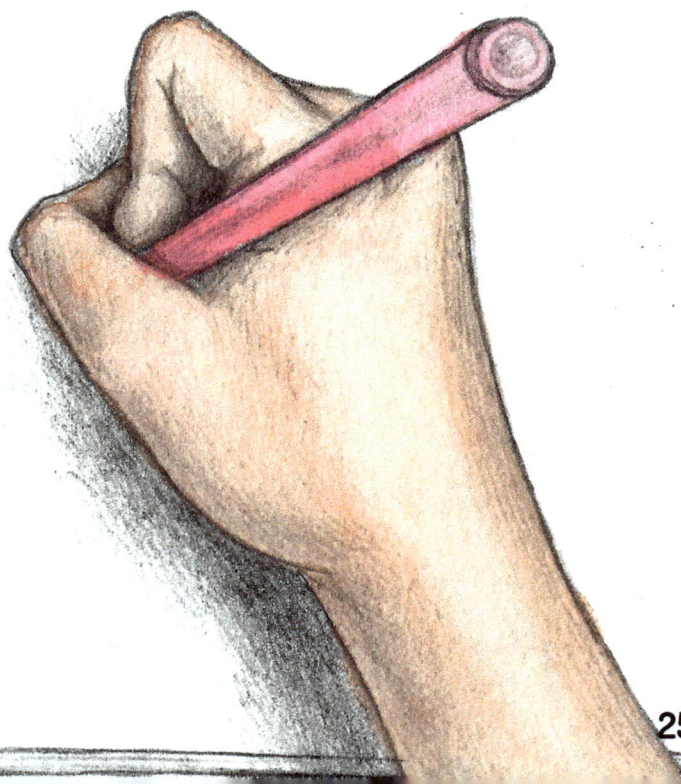

Express YOUR Feelings and YOUR Story!

Hey, it's me, Jamie. I'm here to welcome you to your healing place. This journal has helped me to make sense of my roller coaster of emotions! That's what I want for you.

Draw, write, scribble, or doodle! Write it with love. Draw it to let out the sadness. Scribble or doodle away your anger or frustration. It's all good! What matters on these pages are your feelings. This is not about the cancer diagnosis. This is not about seeing whether or not your cancer journey matches my family's journey. And it certainly is *not* about spelling or if your sentences make sense.

There are NO RULES!

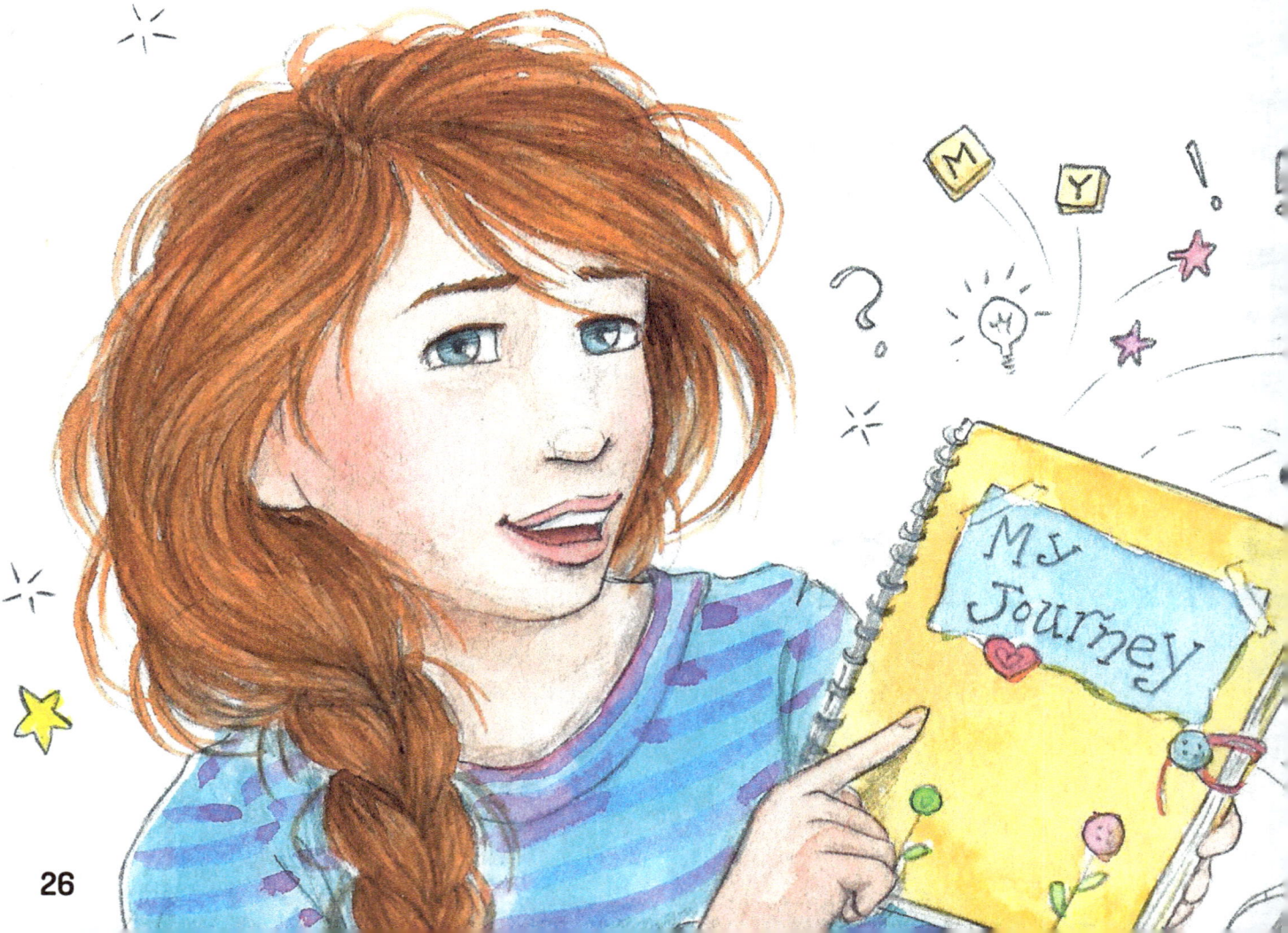

This is all about YOU! It's about your power to define your own reality. You can choose to share or not share. You can reread or add new thoughts. You can delete old ones. Let the prompts be just that . . . words to get you thinking.

Before you begin, I want you to meet Speckles. Speckles has kind of been my security. Speckles is like that old favorite blanket or stuffed animal that you still like to cuddle with late at night or when you just need a friend. Look for Speckles throughout to make you smile!

"Fill your paper with the breathings of your heart."

—William Wordsworth

Worried. Write about a time when you were worried during the cancer journey.

Relieved. Describe what being relieved feels like for you.

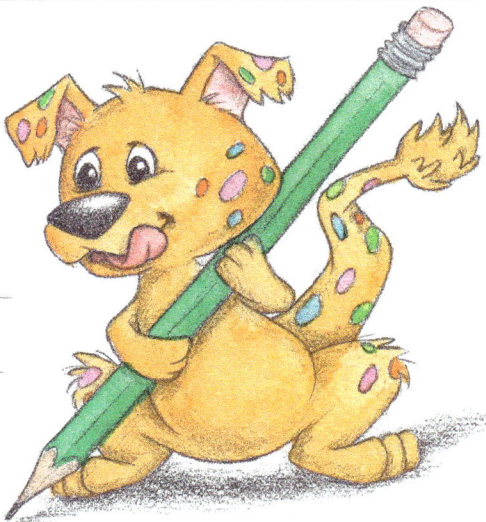

Curious.
Make a list of all the times you were curious. What questions would you still like to ask?

_____

_____

_____

_____

_____

_____

_____

_____

_____

_____

_____

_____

_____

_____

_____

_____

_____

_____

Anger. Anger can look like so many things. How do you express your anger? What colors represent your anger? How did anger cause you pain?

_____

_____

_____

_____

_____

_____

_____

_____

_____

_____

_____

_____

_____

_____

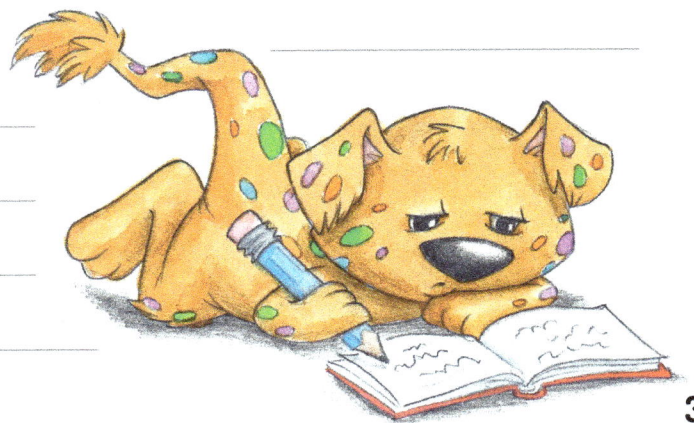

Proud! Show the proud moments!

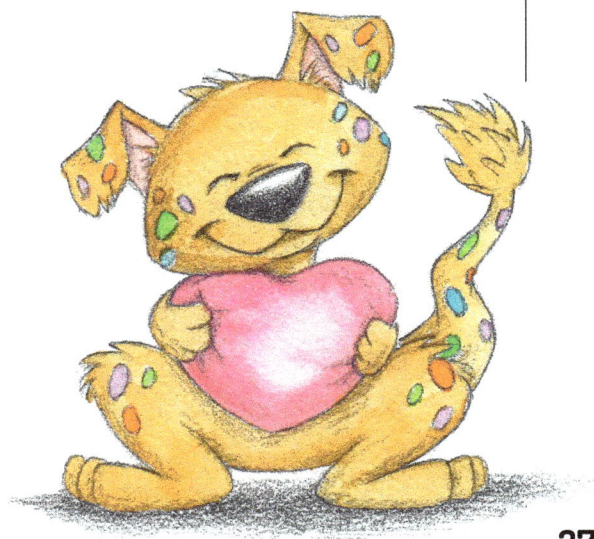

Brave! Me? Yes, I am! Shout it from the rooftops!

Inspiration. What does that mean to you? How has your sibling inspired you? How do you think you've inspired your sibling?

_____

_____

_____

_____

_____

_____

_____

_____

_____

_____

_____

_____

_____

_____

_____

Forgotten? I get that. I felt forgotten when . . .

_____

_____

_____

_____

_____

_____

_____

_____

_____

_____

_____

_____

_____

_____

_____

_____

_____

_____

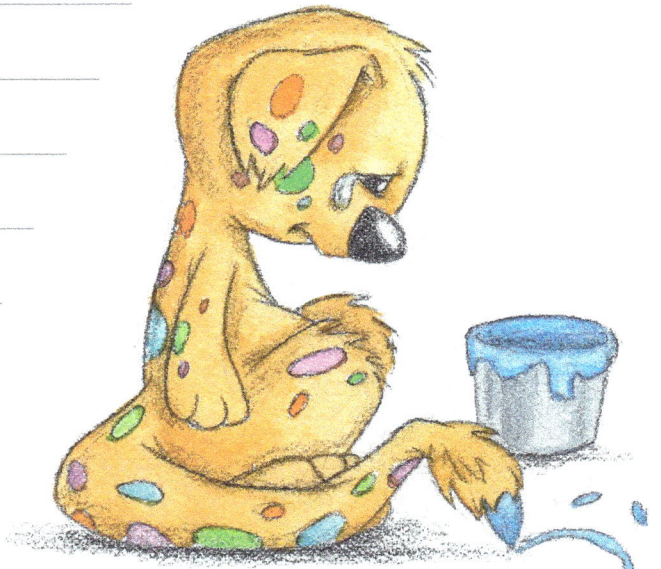

Happy. Show the happy times—in colors or words or with photos.

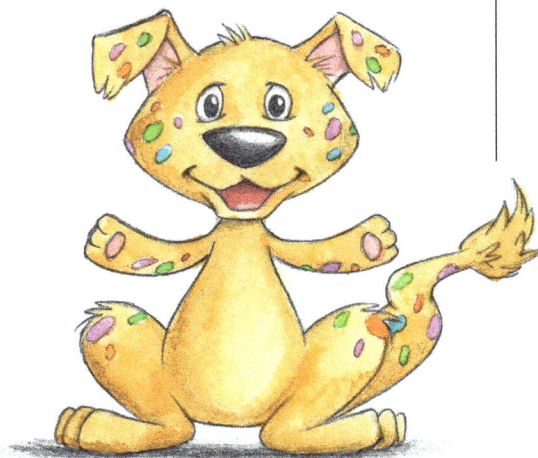

Confusion? There are so many ways to feel confused. What does confusion feel like for you?

_____

_____

_____

_____

_____

_____

_____

_____

_____

_____

_____

_____

_____

_____

_____

_____

_____

Guilt. What's the first thing that popped into your head?

Jealousy. What really made you jealous?

_____

_____

_____

_____

_____

_____

_____

_____

_____

_____

_____

_____

_____

_____

_____

_____

_____

Selfish. Draw it in colors. What does it look like for you?

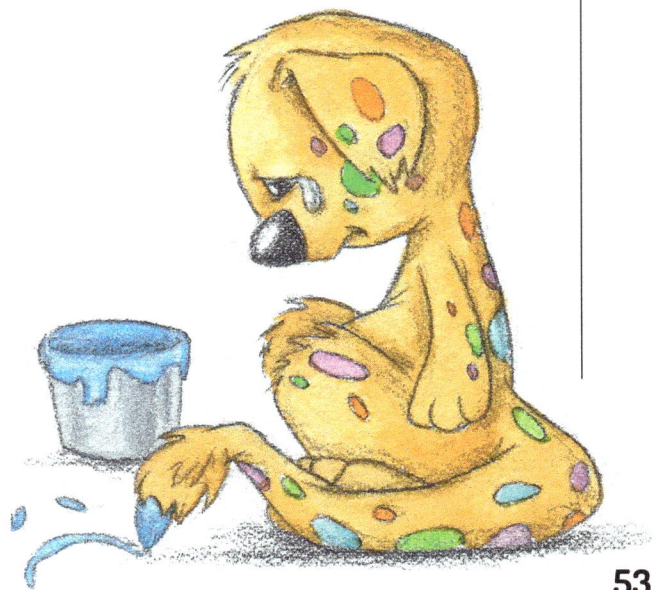

Loved and valued. When? Where? List specific times.
Does a song come to mind?

_____

_____

_____

_____

_____

_____

_____

_____

_____

_____

_____

_____

_____

_____

Speechless. Speckles wants to know about those times. Make a list.

_____

_____

_____

_____

_____

_____

_____

_____

_____

_____

_____

_____

_____

_____

_____

_____

Helpful. Speckles knows you are helpful. Let's see it! List it! Draw it!

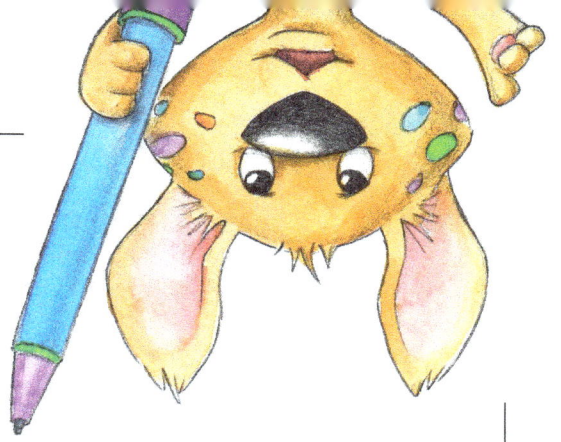

Voice.
Here is one more place for you to use however you want because "your voice matters."

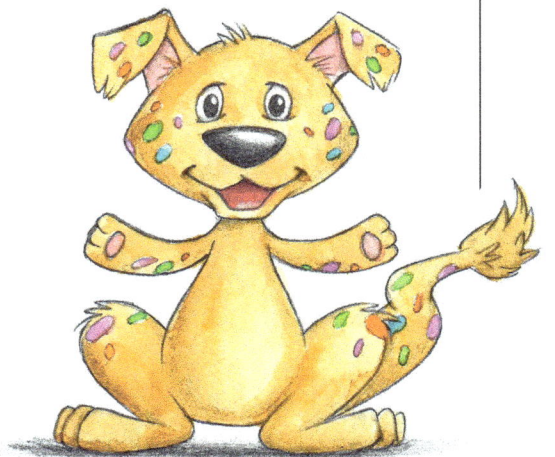

Speckles is here to let you in on a secret!

Art is a powerful way to release your emotions.

Use colored pencils, markers, paint, or whatever medium speaks to you. Remember, don't worry about perfection or creating a masterpiece. Let your heart guide you.

The blank pages that follow are for YOU!
Are you stuck?
Check out the next page for some ideas.

Use bright colors to show anger, jealousy, excitement, or happiness.

Try softer colors to embrace calmness and relief.
Experiment with different lines and shapes.
Sharp, jagged lines can show a sense of worry, being forgotten, angry or frustrated.

Soft curves and lines may show curiosity, being loved, proud, or brave.
Try different textures!
Layer the colors!
Maybe you scribble or just doodle!
NO matter what **YOU** decide to do, this is **FOR YOU!**

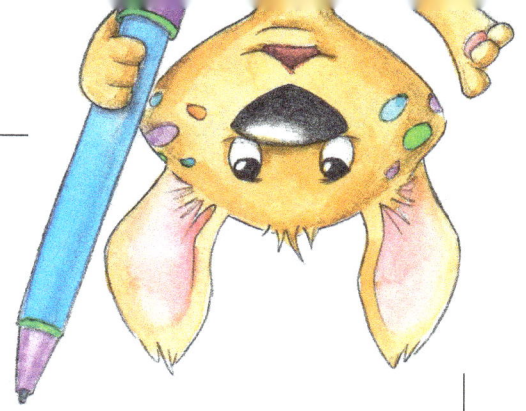

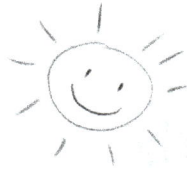

About the author

Sharon Wozny

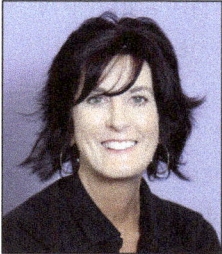

Inspired by her more than three years of volunteering with Children's Cancer Network (CCN), author Sharon Wozny has created a book designed for siblings of pediatric cancer patients. While working with families affected by cancer, Sharon discovered an untapped need among the young people whose entire lives are affected by a sibling's diagnosis. She set out to give these siblings a voice and offer a way for them to help manage the wide range of feelings they might be experiencing. *Jamie's Journey: Cancer from the Voice of a Sibling*, part-book, part-journal, giving young people a safe place to express their emotions. "Siblings of pediatric cancer patients often get lost or forgotten in the throes of the cancer diagnosis," says Wozny. "It's not out of intention, just out of the craziness of what cancer does to a family and the time constraints, worry, angst, and appointments."

Wozny grew up in Massapequa, Long Island and earned a bachelor's degree in elementary education from Oswego State University. She later earned a master's degree in counselor education from Arizona State University. During her thirty-year career in education, Sharon particularly enjoyed teaching her students how to write. As the author of *Jamie's Journey: Cancer from the Voice of a Sibling*, Wozny followed the advice she gave her pupils. "I always taught my students to write what you are passionate about," she said. "If you don't, it won't resonate with people and your true essence won't come through."

Sharon has two grown children, Hailey and Jordan, and lives in Arizona with her husband, Joe.

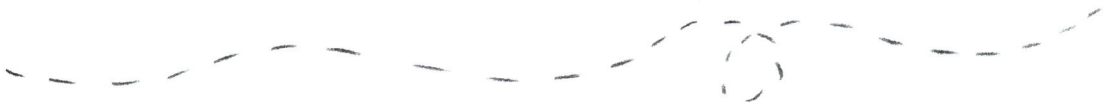

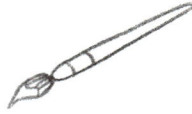

About the illustrator

Melissa Bailey

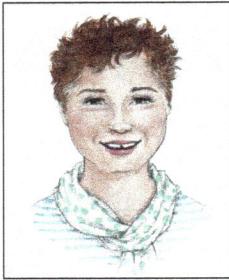

As a child, Melissa Bailey often thought about how cool it would be to illustrate children's books. Many years and thirty-seven books later, her childhood dream is now her real-life job. Melissa felt a special connection to *Jamie's Journey: Cancer from a Voice of a Sibling* because while illustrating this book, her grandma was going through cancer treatments (and happily is in remission now). Surrounded by family, friends, a poodle named Archie, and art supplies, Melissa lives on a dirt road near a small town in Michigan.

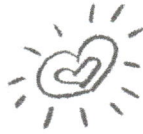

*"**Jamie's Journey** is the best medicine for siblings of kids with cancer. With comforting text and gorgeous illustrations, it gently explores the sometimes difficult emotions that arise in siblings ... This book is a gem!"*

— Nancy Keene, author of 14 books for families of children with cancer, alexslemonade.org/childhood-cancer/guides

*"I'm a sibling whose sister has cancer. It was really helpful to read about someone whose sibling also has cancer, even if it is a fictional character. **Jamie's Journey** helps kids deal with their feelings such as jealousy and guilt. It is my #1 children's cancer book recommendation."*

— Abby, age 10

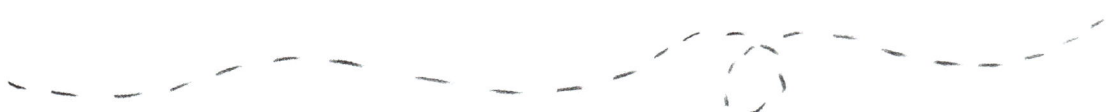

CHiLdREn's
cancer network

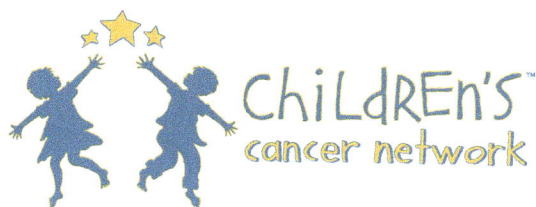

When I began attending Children's Cancer Network's fashion show nine years ago, little did I know how this organization would capture my heart and become such an integral part of my life. From the Luttrells, to the courageous families, to the dedicated volunteers working tirelessly to give hope, CCN is an inspiration!

Most importantly, I would not have been inspired to write this book.

Steve and Patti Luttrell have experienced firsthand the effects of childhood cancer. Their son Jeff, now twenty-seven, was diagnosed at age five with leukemia. Desiring to make a difference for families, Jeff's older sister, Jenny, organized the first fashion show to raise money and thirteen years later, the legacy continues! Earning a degree in graphic design, Jeff has focused his energy on healing through art and creativity. He provided the inspiration for the character of Speckles in my book.

Children's Cancer Network supports families throughout their cancer journey with programs designed to provide financial assistance, promote education, encourage healthy lifestyles, build self-esteem, and create awareness of the issues they face related to childhood cancer.

Understanding the unique struggles that siblings face during these uncertain times, CCN provided financial support to publishing *Jamie's Journey*. Humbly, I thank the Luttrells and the board of directors for acknowledging the positive impact this book will have on families affected by cancer.

For more information about Children's Cancer Network, visit www.childrenscancernetwork.org or call 480-398-1564.

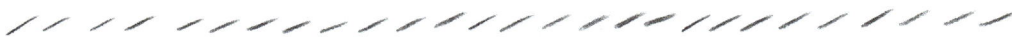

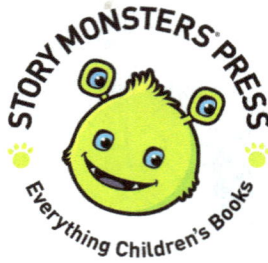

About the publisher

Story Monsters Press

Story Monsters Press is an award-winning, full-service children's book publisher dedicated to stories that inspire, celebrate diversity, and build character. Each book includes an activities guide, making it a valuable resource for parents and educators.

Founded by Linda F. Radke in 1985, we've grown from Five Star Publications into a nationally recognized publishing house, honored for our excellence in book marketing and author support.

We guide authors at every stage—from concept to publication—offering expert editorial, design, and distribution services. Our marketing solutions help books stand out and reach wider audiences.

With our exclusive Little Monster Read-Along program, we bring stories to life through professional narration, offering young readers an engaging, immersive experience.

At Story Monsters Press, you're not just publishing a book—you're joining a passionate community devoted to storytelling and literacy.

Ready to get started?

Contact Linda at 480-940-8182 or email Linda@StoryMonsters.com

Explore more at StoryMonsters.com

Celebrate the power of storytelling—with Story Monsters Press.